Toothache at Big Mouth Bend

TOOTHACHE AT BIG MOUTH BEND

BY

Tracy Carol Taylor

Toothache At Big Mouth Bend

This is a work of fiction. Names, characters, places, and incidents either are the product of the author's imagination or are used fictitiously, and any resemblance to actual persons, living or dead, businesses establishments, events, or locales is entirely coincidental. The publisher does not have any control over and does not assume any responsibility for author or third-party websites or their contents.

Prince of Pages Inc.

N. Carlin Springs Road.

Arlington, VA 22203

www.princeofpages.com

ISBN: 978-1-9492522-0-0

Cover Art by Christine Tu

Contents

Chapter 1

Once upon a time, a long time ago, there was the valley of Big Mouth Bend. Big Mouth Bend had a lush landscape of celery trees and spinach grass. Clear blue skies and wide open prairie. In the middle of this lush valley was the town of Gumm. Its people were happy and prosperous. Sheriff T. Paste kept the little town orderly and clean. But... every once in a while...

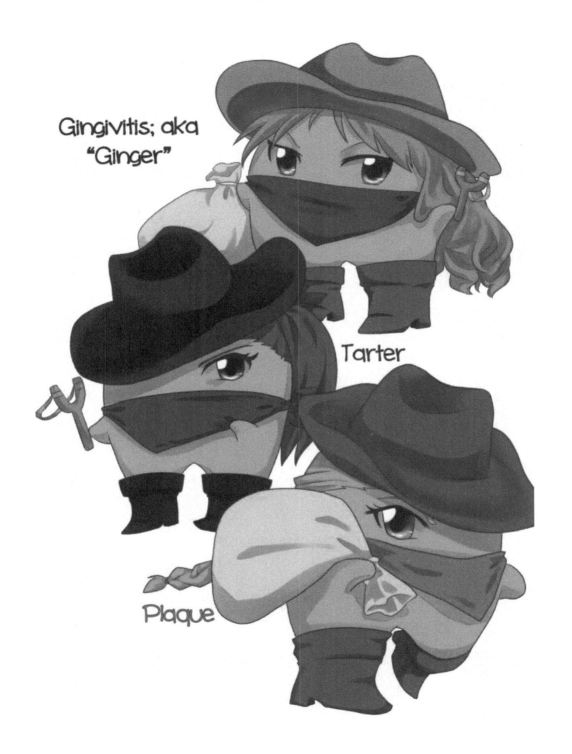

Gingivitis; aka "Ginger"

Tarter

Plaque

"Sheriff! Sheriff! You gotta come quick the Cavity Gang is at it again. They just robbed the town bank and got away with 500 enamels." cried the town banker.

"Don't worry none Mr. White. I'll get 'em." assured Sheriff Paste.

So, the Sheriff rode out on his horse and chased down the Cavity Gang. Ginger, Tarter, and Plaque were female triplets and they were always causing trouble. They didn't like the town of Gumm. It was just too clean for their taste. Usually, they just dug holes in peoples' lawns, and graffitied the walls; but robbing the 1st Baby Tooth Bank was just plain low down.

Sheriff Paste soon caught up with them. He recovered the money and chased the Cavity Gang away. Sheriff Paste was greeted by a warm and cheering crowd, as he rode back into town with the town's money.

"Here ya go Mr. White. Just like I promised." smiled Sheriff Paste, as he handed the money back to Mr. White.

"Thank you, Sheriff. You are a true credit to this community." praised Mr. White.

"Aw twer'nt nothing." laughed the Sheriff.

"Sheriff he's right. Without you around, the Cavity Gang would turn this town to rot." commended Mayor Molar, as he patted the sheriff on the back. "Come on down to the saloon and let me buy you a drink."

"Sure thing, Mayor. It'd be my honor." accepted Sheriff Paste.

The bartender, Braces, greeted them as they came in the door.

"Hey Braces, give the Sheriff a shot of the new stuff." recommended Mr. White.

"New Stuff? You mean there's something new besides water and milk in this here bar?" asked Sheriff Paste.

"Sure is. But it's powerful stuff. So be careful." warned Mr. White.

"Here you go Sheriff." said Braces, as he gave the Sheriff his drink.

Sheriff Paste looked at the drink.

"It's yellow." he said.

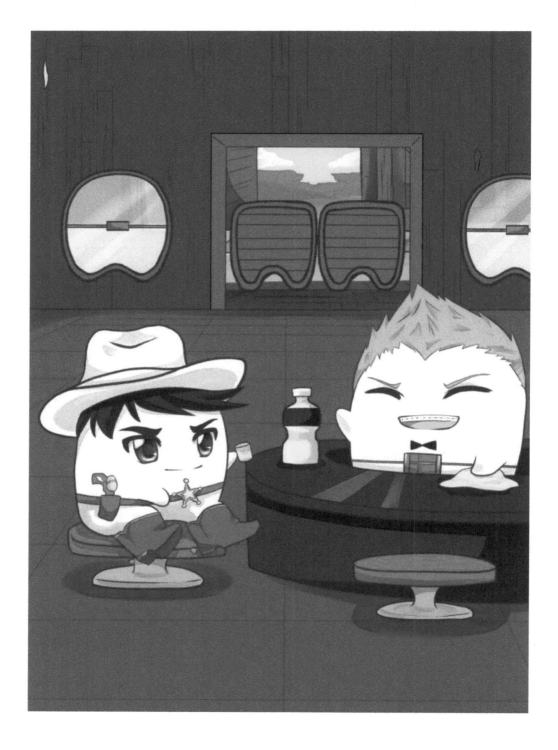

"Might be, but it sure ain't cowardly. Go on try it." said Mr. White.

Sheriff sniffed at it first. It even smelled strong. Then he took a sip. It set his mouth on fire.

"Oh Boy! That stuff will kick you in the teeth. What's it called?" complained Sheriff Paste.

"Lysterine." chuckled Braces. "That there is the drink of Men."

"Or something to take the paint off of fences." choked Sheriff Paste.

"Ha ha ha ha." they laughed.

And so it was, in the town of Gumm. Law and Order ruled the day. But that was all about to change.

Chapter 2

It was a dark and moonless night when the Cavity Gang visited Farmer Carnivore's Ranch. They snuck in all quiet like and went straight for the barn.

"Shhh, nice and quiet now girls. Get them cows loaded." whispered Ginger.

"I don't get it, Ginger." questioned Tartar. "Why are we stealing cows?"

"Boss said to get the cows because we failed to get the money from the bank. Boss says we need capital." explained Ginger.

"We got a capital." said Tartar. "The city of Roots ain't that far away."

"Not that kind of capital, dummy." scolded Ginger.

"You girls quit jaw'n and load them cows up." ordered Plaque.

"Quit your nagging Plak. We're almost done." said Ginger.

And so, in the middle of the night, the Cavity Gang made off with all the cows.

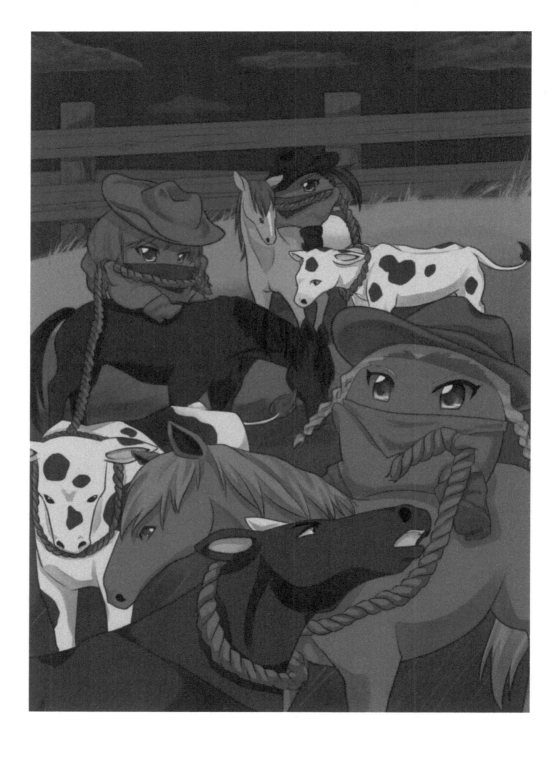

The next morning, the townspeople awoke to a big and terrible surprise.

"Sheriff! Sheriff! It's horrible!" exclaimed Farmer Carnivore.

"What's the matter Carny? What's wrong?" asked the Sheriff.

"The cows...they're gone! Somebody done stole all our cows!" cried Farmer Carnivore.

"No cows means no milk." reasoned the Sheriff. "Who would do such a thing?"

"You know who. It was the Cavity Gang. They're the only bad in this town." said Farmer Carnivore.

"You don't know that." said the Sheriff. "Did anybody see them do it?"

"Course not. It happened in the middle of the night. We was all sleeping. But I know it was them, I can feel it in my bones." accused Farmer Carnivore.

"Alright. I'll look into it." promised Sheriff Paste. "I'll go and have a talk with them."

"O.K. Sheriff. I'll trust you to get my cows back." relented Farmer Carnivore.

So, Sheriff Paste went on over to the Cavity

Gang's hide out. It was a cave on the west side of the mountain.

"Anybody home?!" he called out.

"Well, well ain't this nice. Hey girls, the Sheriff's come a calling." announced Plaque.

"I knew you'd warn up to me sooner or later, Sheriff." said Ginger.

"Hi Sheriff." smiled Tartar.

"Howdy Miss Tartar." greeted Sheriff Paste, politely.

"You want some refreshment." offered Ginger. "Seeing as you came all this way to see us. I'd be impolite not to offer you something."

"No thank you, Miss Ginger. I'm here to ask you about some missing cows." said Sheriff Paste.

"Missing Cows?" smirked Plaque. "No cows around here."

"You're welcome to search my room." offered Ginger coyly.

"Uh, no thank you. I think I'll just have a look around outside." said Sheriff Paste, as he backed away from Ginger.

"Go ahead." said Plaque. "We ain't got them."

"Feel free to come back anytime Sheriff." said

Ginger, as she waved goodbye. "You can arrest me any day."

Sheriff Paste left their cave home and searched the grounds outside. But he found no trace of the cows; and nothing that would suggest that the girls had left the cave last night. Their wash was still hanging on the line drying. So, Sheriff Paste headed back to town.

Since he didn't find any clues at the Cavity Gang's place, He decided to go to Farmer Carnivore's Ranch to look for clues.

He looked in the fields where the cows ate. He looked in the barn where the cows slept. But he could find no clues as to who took the cows. So, he returned to town. But when he got there he was in for another surprise.

"Come one and come all. Try the new drink that's sweeping the nation. It will quench your thirst! It's cold and it's cool. It will even make you feel good! Have a SODA and a smile!" called FruCose.

"Who are they?" asked Sheriff Paste.

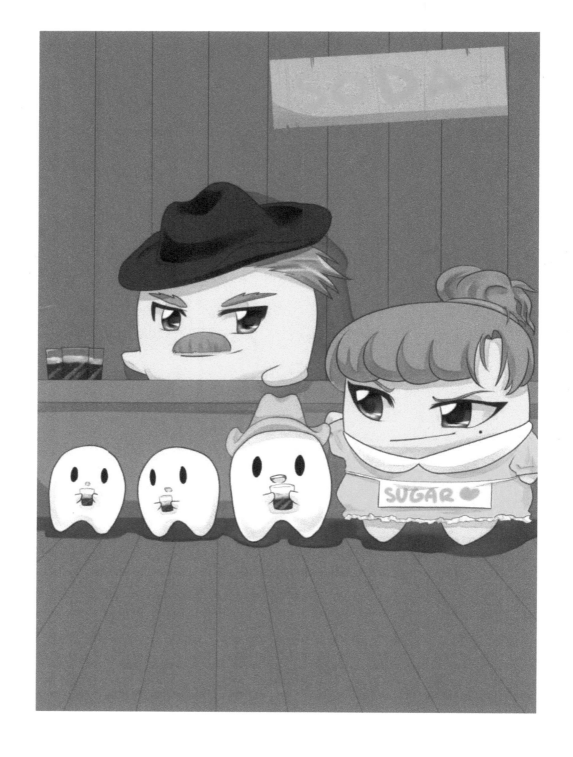

"That's FruCose and his sister Lady Sugar. They just opened up a new store in town. They're even given away free drinks." explained Mayor Molar.

"Well ain't that something. I hope it tastes better than that Lysterine stuff you gave me." teased Sheriff Paste.

"Indeed, it does." said Mayor Molar. "Go and see for yourself."

Sheriff Paste watched as curious parents gathered around to look at the new drink; but it was the kids that really took a shine to the new drink. They just couldn't seem to get enough of it.

"It's seems mighty peculiar that our cows should disappear one day and these guys show up the next." reasoned Sheriff Paste.

"Maybe, but there's no law against selling goods and services." reminded Mayor Molar.

"Believe me mayor, this is more than coincidence. I got a bad feeling about this." said Sheriff Paste.

"Well, until you can prove it. There's nothing you can do, is there?" said Mayor Molar.

Chapter 3

And so, the town of Gumm got a new drink, SODA. But all was not as it seemed and soon the real danger of soda was revealed.

Soon the doctor's office was full of sick kids.

"Doctor! Doctor! My little boy is sick! He's got a toothache." called Father Denture.

"Put him in the bed, over there, with the others." said the Doctor Floss.

"Are all these children sick?" asked Father Denture.

"Yes. It seems we have an epidemic on our hands." said Doctor Floss, sadly. "I've called for a specialist to help out. He should be arriving on the next train."

"Well what do we do in the mean time?" asked Father Denture.

"Well, I'll give them a good brushing of fluoride and hope that the sugar rush wears off." said Doctor Floss. "But I want to keep him here with the others for observation."

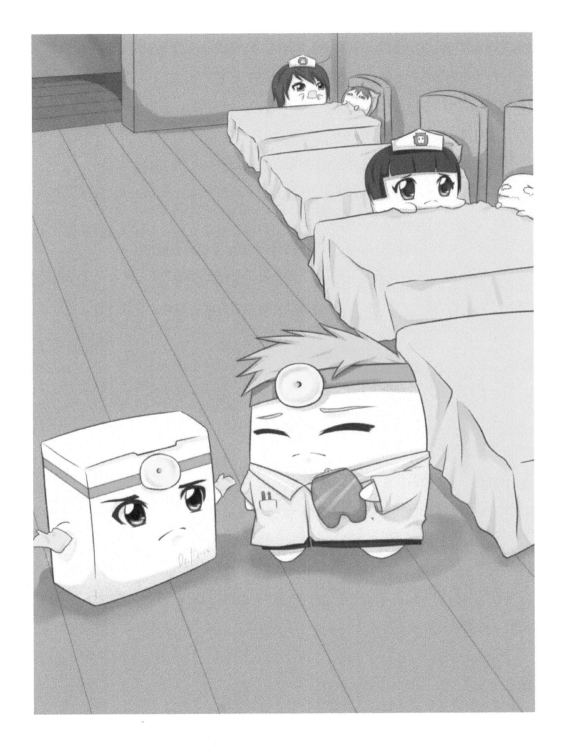

Meanwhile, Ginger strolled into town wearing a new dress. She passed right by the Sheriff's office. Sheriff Paste was sitting on his porch watching her pass by.

"Morning, Sheriff." she greeted, brightly.

"Morning, Miss Ginger." he answered. "That sure is a pretty dress."

"Why thank you, sheriff." she smiled.

"Where'd you get the money?" he asked. "You're not robbing banks again, are you?"

"No." said Ginger. "I got the money from my job."

"Job?" he asked.

"Yes, I work down at the Soda Shop." she answered.

"Hm. That's mighty convenient. You still insisting that you and your sisters had nothing to do with those missing cows?" he asked.

"Yes, sir. I do." said Ginger.

"Alright, But I got my eye on you. All of you." he warned.

"Have a nice day, sheriff." said Ginger, as she left.

"The trains here!" called an energetic boy, as he ran by.

Sheriff Paste got up and went to greet the train. He met Doctor Floss at the station.

"Heard you're waiting for a specialist." said Sheriff Paste.

"Yes, this epidemic has me baffled." admitted Doctor Floss. "He should be on this train."

Both men waited. People got on and off, but none of them were a specialist. Soon a man got off the train, and he was carrying a Bow Staff Toothbrush. He walked right up to Doctor Floss and Sheriff Paste.

"I hear your looking for a specialist." he said.

"Yes." said Doctor Floss. "And you are?"

"Doctor Lo Fang, PHD in dentistry and a black belt martial artist." he bowed. "I am at your service."

"Boy am I glad you're here." said Doctor Floss. "We've got a bad epidemic."

"Let me check your data." said Dr. Fang. "And I'll see what I can do."

"Yes, of course this way." escorted Doctor Floss.

The Doctor Floss took Dr. Fang to his clinic and showed him his data and his patients. Dr. Fang examined each one and then asked...

"What have they been eating or drinking?"

"Well, we've no milk anymore. Someone stole our cows. So, we've got water, soda, and Lysterine; but since you've got to be over eighteen to drink that Lysterine. I recon the kids have been drinking that new-fangled drink, soda." explained Doctor Floss.

"Hm. New shop, just opened." reasoned Dr. Fang.

"That's right. Been open a month now." said Doctor Floss. "The place is always full of kids."

"You didn't have this problem when they were drinking milk, did you?" asked Dr. Fang.

"No." answered Doctor Floss.

"It's Sugar Rot; the soda is making your kids sick. The chemical compound is high in sugar and salt. As you can see, it's not good for you. Have these kids drink nothing but water and they'll be fine." reported Dr. Fang.

"That's not going to be easy. That soda stuff tastes real good." said Doctor Floss.

"If they don't stop drinking it, the problem will only get worse. In the meantime, I'm going to see your sheriff about your missing cows." said Dr. Fang.

So, Dr. Fang went to see Sheriff Paste.

"Afternoon, Dr. Fang." greeted Sheriff Paste.

"Good afternoon sheriff." said Dr. Fang.

"Did you find out what's making our kids sick?" asked Sheriff Paste.

"It's the soda." said Dr. Fang.

"I knew that stuff was no good." said Sheriff Paste.

"Tell me Sheriff, has Lady Sugar shone her face?" asked Dr. Fang.

"No. But her brother FruCose runs the soda shop. He's even got the Cavity Gang working for him. And I didn't think anything could reform those girls." said Sheriff Paste.

"Sheriff, I'm here to offer my help in finding those missing cows. I think Lady Sugar has them. And if we don't get those cows back and get these kids drinking milk again. Things are only going to get worse." explained Dr. Fang.

"Worse? How could things get worse?" asked Sheriff Paste.

"You see Lady Sugar doesn't work alone. Gumm D. Seas and his little sister Tuth D. Kay will soon follow. Soda makes some people hyper, makes some people lazy, and makes everyone fat. If we don't stop her now, this town will go rotten to the core." explained Dr. Fang.

"Sheriff, you gotta come quick! Some kids are playing chicken on horseback! They're standing on the horse's back and the first one to fall is chicken!" reported Mr. Tongue.

"Sheriff, you've gotta come and stop the kids from breaking the windows down at the school!" reported Ms. Dentine.

"Sheriff, we need you to stop Cody and Jessie from climbing trees in Rotten Wood!" reported Mr. Pulp.

"You see Sheriff, it's already started." said Dr. Fang.

"You'll help me?" asked Sheriff Paste.

"All I can." assured Dr. Fang.

"Then let's go." said Sheriff Paste.

Chapter 4

By sundown, the jailhouse was full of kids. The Sheriff gave them nothing but water to drink and by morning they were calmed down enough to go home. So, he let them all go, into the custody of their parents, with a warning to stop drinking that soda.

But they didn't listen and after another week of arresting kids doing stupid stuff, the Sheriff was looking forward to a drink of Listerine. Sheriff Paste walked into the saloon and fell into a seat at the bar.

"What's the matter Sheriff, you don't look so good." commented Braces.

"I'm tired Braces." said Sheriff Paste. "These kids are running wild."

"Yep, I recon they are." said Braces, as he cleaned a glass.

"I've got to find those cows, but I've got no clues. I don't know what to do." admitted Sheriff Paste.

All of a sudden, the sheriff heard gunfire.

"Now what?!" He dreaded.

"Pay attention all you losers. My name's Gumm D. Seas and this here is my little sister Tuth D. Kay. And from now on we own this town." announced Gumm loudly.

"Recon I got something to say about that." said Sheriff Paste, standing up to them.

"Well looky here, Tuth." said Gumm, as a wicked smile spread across his face. "We got the law to come and greet us."

"What's up Law man?" asked Tuth.

"You two can leave our town." warned Sheriff Paste, with a scowl. "We don't need your kind here."

"Our kind?" chuckled Tuth. "Gumm, I think we've been insulted."

"Yeah, I'm feeling real unwelcome." smirked Gumm. "Alright, Sheriff we'll leave your town...in pieces."

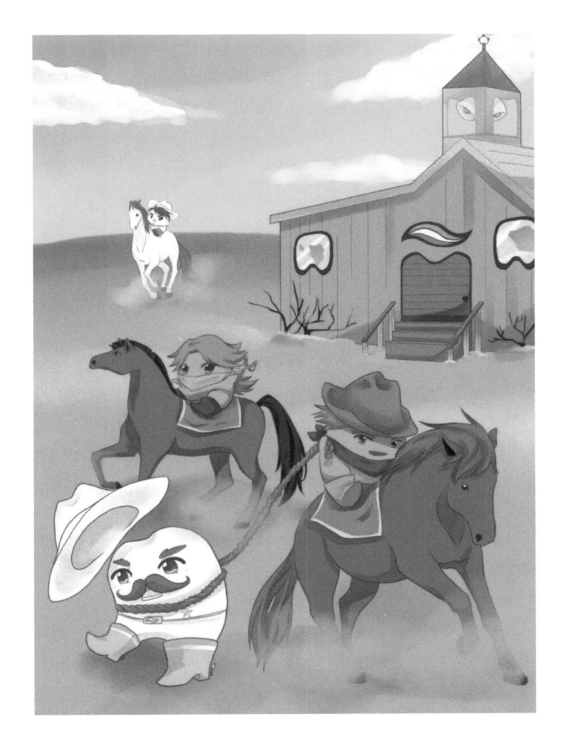

That's when Gumm D. Seas and Tuth D. Kay started tearing up the town. They set the Jaw Bone home store on fire, shot out all the windows of the church, and dragged Mayor Molar through the street behind their horses.

Sheriff Paste and Dr. Fang confronted them. Sheriff Paste lassoed Tuth with his dental floss lasso. And Dr. Fang brushed off Gumm with his martial arts bow staff toothbrush. Soon Sheriff Paste had Gumm and his sister Tuth behind bars.

Tuth lay on the bed and looked up at the ceiling, while her brother taunted the Sheriff.

"What are you smiling at?" asked Sheriff Paste.

"You know cows are real tasty when you fry them and slap them between two buns." smirked Gumm.

"Hmm, stop it you're making me hungry. We ain't eat yet." complained Tuth. "Hey Sheriff, when's dinner?"

"Well, on tonight's menu is salad with a light vinaigrette and water with a twist of lemon." said Sheriff Paste.

"Oh, God, I'm gonna die." whined Tuth.

"Don't worry little sister. Once our lawyer gets

us out, I'll treat you to a nice juicy hamburger." said Gumm. "Too bad you don't have any cows Sheriff. You could make us a real nice meal."

"Fried burgers? That just ain't natural." told Sheriff Paste. "Good beef should be grilled to perfection."

Suddenly, a gut feeling hit Sheriff Paste right in his ...gut.

"You two wouldn't know anything about Farmer Carnivore's missing cows, would you?" asked Sheriff Paste.

"What cows?" smirked Gumm.

"Right. Dr. Fang watch our prisoners for me. I'll be right back." said Sheriff Paste.

The Sheriff soon came back carrying two buckets.

"Is that what I think it is?" asked Dr. Fang.

"Yep." said Sheriff Paste.

"If I were you two, I'd start confessing." warned Dr. Fang, with a knowing grin.

"And if we don't?" asked Tuth.

That's when Sheriff Paste tossed the bucket of Lysterine on them.

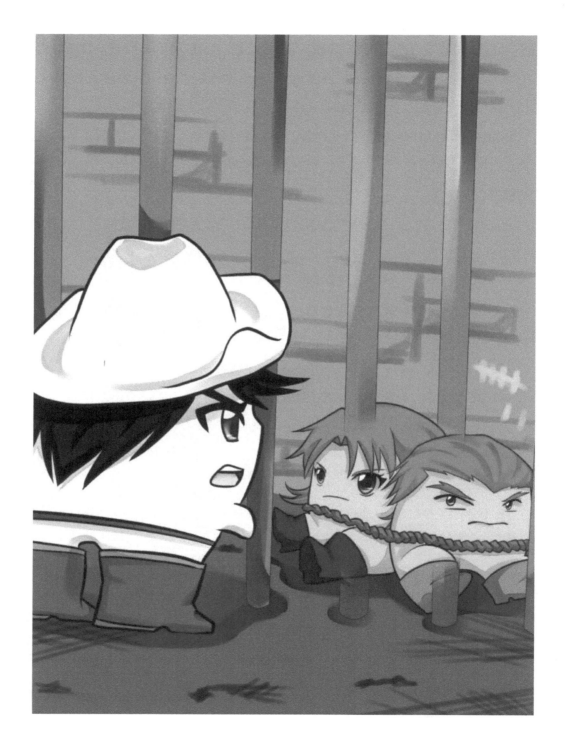

"Jumping Jehoshaphat!!" screamed Gumm. "What is that stuff?! It burns like a bad sunburn!!"

"Now you two want to start talking. I've got one more bucket and a whole saloon full of this stuff." threatened Sheriff Paste.

The two said nothing; they just looked at each other. So Sheriff Paste tossed the other bucket of Lysterine on them.

"O.K! O.K! Just stop throwing that stuff on us!" hollered Tuth.

That's when they told the Sheriff everything. Lady Sugar paid the Cavity Gang to steal Farmer Carnivore's cows. Then she sent her brother FruCose to set up shop here. They were planning to take the cows back East and open up a fast food restaurant. The cows were being shipped out on the midnight train from the capital city Roots.

With a signed confession from Gumm D. Seas and Tuth D. Kay, Sheriff Paste closed down the soda shop and arrested the Cavity Gang. With them safely in jail, he and Dr. Fang hurried to reach the town of Roots.

It was an hour to midnight when they arrived

in the city of Roots. FruCose and his gang met them at the city limits.

"I know'd you be here when I saw you arrest D. Seas and his little sister Tuth." said FruCose.

"Give up FruCose and return our Cows!" ordered Sheriff Paste.

"Give up? You must be kiddn'. As soon as my sister makes that train, we'll be rich. We'll own you and every city in Big Mouth Bend." said FruCose.

"Can't let you make that train." said Sheriff Paste.

"And I can't let you stop us." said FruCose. "Get 'em boys."

Sheriff Paste got into a shootout with Buck Tooth and the Molar Gang; while Dr. Fang took on FruCose and Corn Syrup in a martial arts battle.

The bad guys fought hard, but the good guys fought harder and soon Sheriff Paste and Dr. Fang had all the bad guys rounded up.

Chapter 5

Now there was only one more villain to face, Lady Sugar.

They went to the train station to confront Lady Sugar. Lady Sugar had all the cows loaded and was about to board the train, when Sheriff Paste called out her name.

"Lady Sugar!" he hollered.

Lady Sugar stopped and turned to face them.

"So, you boys made it in time after all. State what you want...quickly...I have a train to catch." she taunted.

"Return our cows!" demanded Sheriff Paste.

"Sorry, no can do. Those cows have a date with a grill back East." explained Lady Sugar.

"Give up, Lady Sugar." ordered Dr. Fang. "We out number you two to one."

"Well Doctor, as I always say, fight fire with fire." she sneered.

Lady Sugar struck a match and dropped it. Suddenly, a wall of fire stood between them and

Lady Sugar. Lady Sugar just laughed as she boarded the train and took off.

"We gotta put out this fire!" said the Sheriff.

So, with the help of Dr. Fang and some of the local townspeople, the fire at the train station was put out.

"We'll never catch her now." feared Dr. Fang.

"Oh, yes we will. She still has to get through Wisdom Tooth Pass. We'll cut her off there." explained Sheriff Paste.

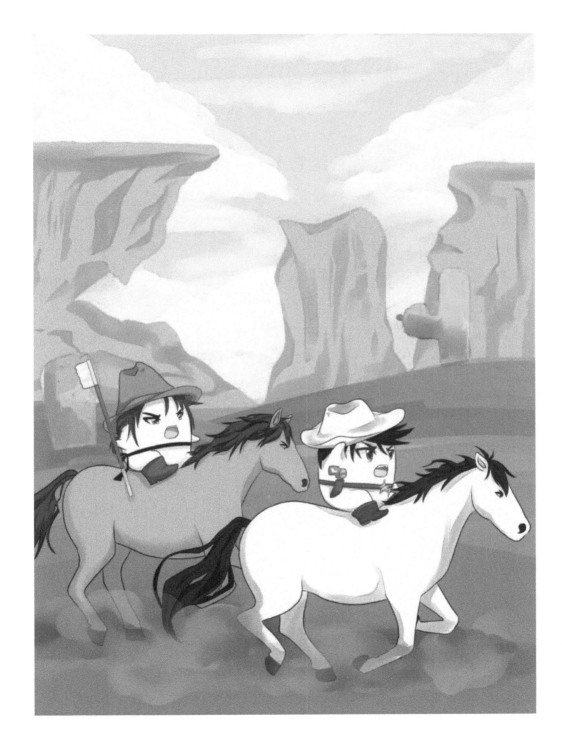

So, Sheriff Paste and Dr. Lo Fang rode their horses hard and fast. They caught up to Lady Sugar's train, passed it, and rode for the Turnoff.

At the turnoff, Sheriff Paste and Dr. Fang pulled the 'switch track' lever. Soon Lady Sugar's train was headed in a new direction.

"Where does this switch off lead?" asked Dr. Fang.

"To Big Gulp Mine." said Sheriff Paste. "She's got nowhere to go."

"I've been waiting a long time to put Lady Sugar out of business." said Dr. Fang.

Aboard the Train, Lady Sugar noticed that something was wrong.

"What the..? This is the wrong direction." she worried.

Lady Sugar went to the first car and looked out of the window. Up ahead, she saw the Mine and the "End of the Line" signal. Soon, the train began to slow down to a stop.

"Dang, this is not good. Engineer, what happened?" she asked, as she made her way over to him.

"Someone used the 'switch track' lever." explained the Engineer.

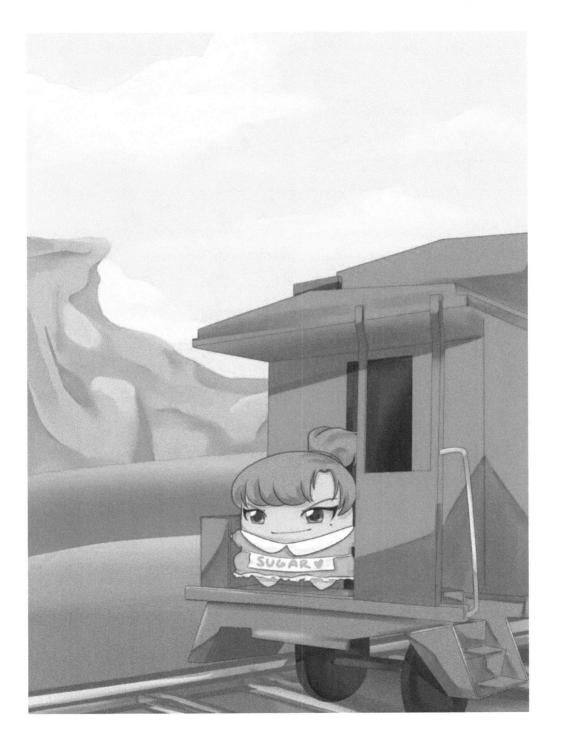

Then she saw Sheriff Paste and Dr. Fang waiting for her.

"I should have known." she growled.

"Give it up Little Lady. You've nowhere left to go." said Sheriff Paste.

Lady Sugar put her hands up and got off the train.

"You won this round, Sheriff. But someday the city of Gumm will be mine." she sneered.

The sheriff moved forward to put the cuffs on her. She waited until he was real close, and then she punched him and knocked him down. Dr. Fang moved to stop her, but she scared his horse. The horse reared up and threw Dr. Fang off his back and to the ground. Lady Sugar mounted the Sheriff's horse and rode away.

"Till next time, Sheriff!" she laughed, as she raced away.

Dr. Fang got up and then helped Sheriff Paste to stand up.

"Should we go after her?" he asked.

"Naw, let her go. We got what we came for. We've got our cows back." said Sheriff Paste.

"You know she'll be back." warned Dr. Fang.

"Yep. But that's O.K. Now we know what she

looks like, we'll keep a look out for her." assured the Sheriff.

So, the City of Gumm got their cows back; much to the excitement and joy of Farmer Carnivore. The children went back to drinking milk and the epidemic of sugar rot was cured.

However, the children still craved SODA. So now the schoolteacher, Professor Crown, gave the children classes on the proper care of their teeth and the dangers of Lady Sugar.

And so, the citizens of Gumm lived happily ever after.

THE END

Other books by Tracy Carol Taylor

CPSIA information can be obtained
at www.ICGtesting.com
Printed in the USA
JSHW050531200223
37886JS00002B/31